EAT BETTER, LIVE BETTER
Nutrition Magazine

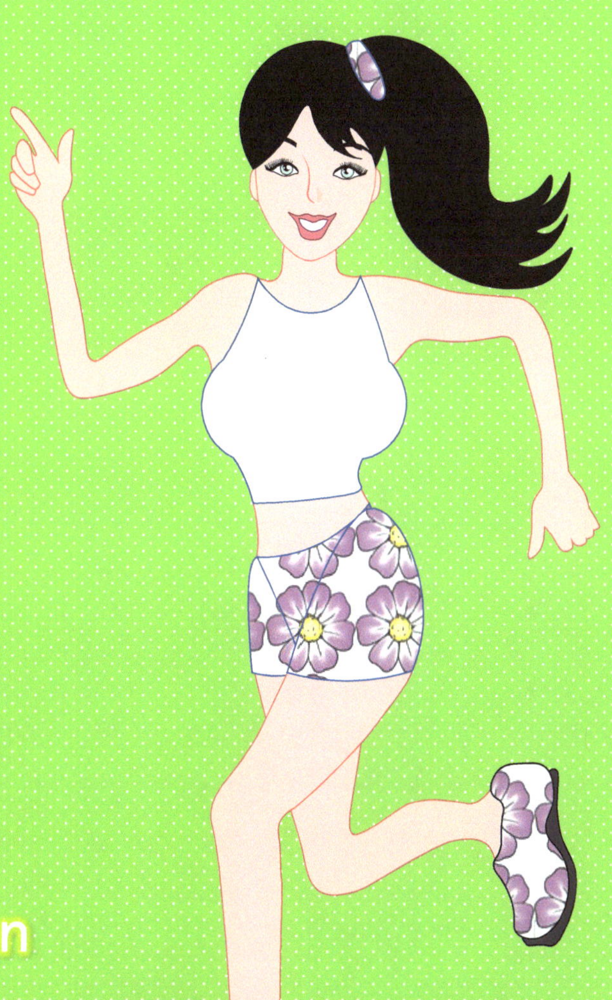

Define
Nutrition

Nutritional
Demands

The Digestion

Strengthening the
inmune system

Food Properties

Healthy
salads

Food
Pyramid
(OMS)

Diet to lose
weight
Week 1

Learn to
combine
foods

AF478779

Destroying my human side in order to be happy

Novel written by Gladys Méndez. Spanish version for sale on Amazon. English version, for sale at Barnes and Nobles.

It is the story of a Colombian woman, who is forced to leave behind her whole life, her children, her family, everything she loves and knows, to travel to a completely unknown country in search of a better future. But that trip will not turn out as she believed, and it will not be what she was looking for. This woman will have to break her heart to pieces to find the true value of her life. She will have to learn with great pain, that mistakes are paid for with blood and that humanity is not what she believed.

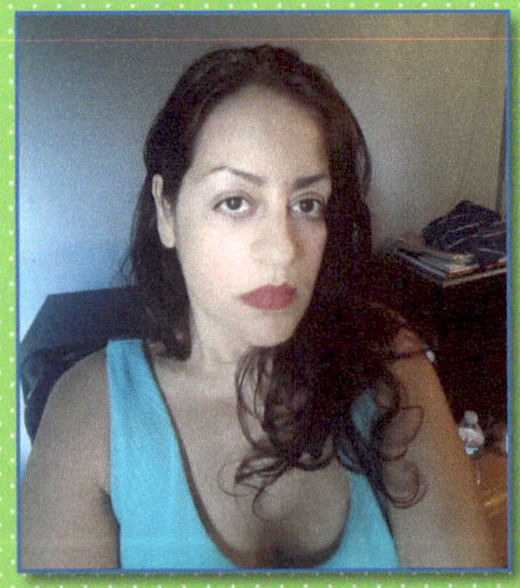

Gladys Méndez: She was born in Yolombó, Antioquia, Colombia. She is a writer for Corazón. Shows interest not only in writing, but also in drawings and the study of nutrition in human beings.

She wrote five books but has only published one. Specialist in Adobe programs, web page design, etc.

You can place your orders through the email mmgy777@Gmail.com

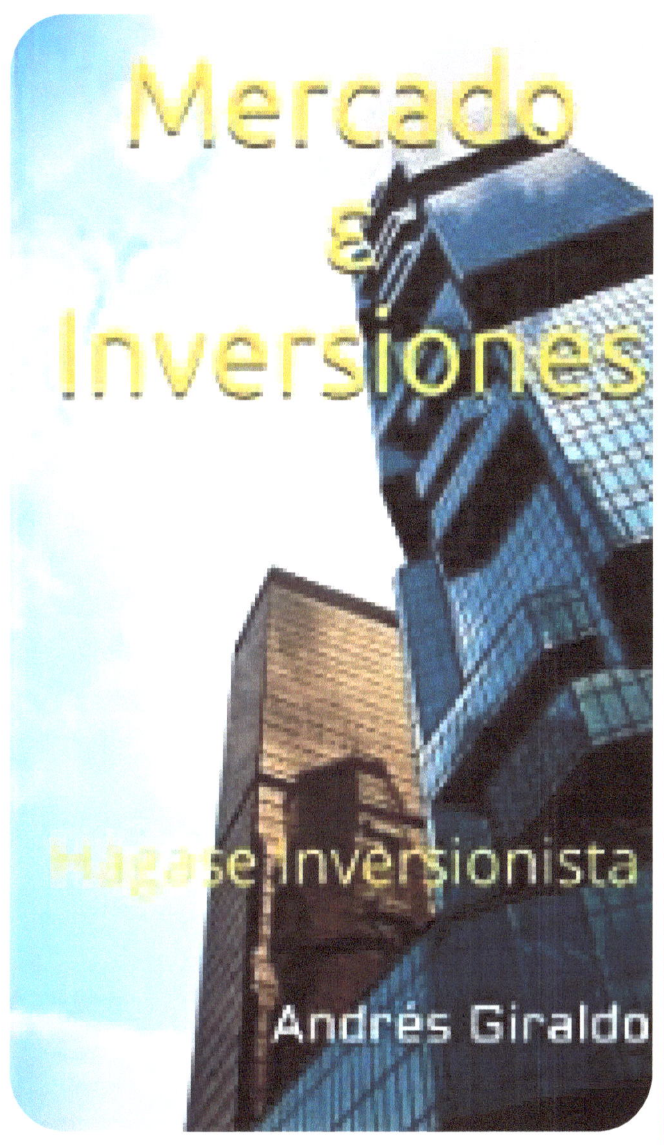

Andrés Felipe Giraldo

He was born in Medellín, Colombia. He grew up in a working family, his father is a philosopher and his mother an accountant, from a very young age he was curious about science and mathematics in general, he had the opportunity to study economics at one of the best universities in his country, at which time he acquired a critical and analytical sense of the economic and financial environment; Later, his experience as a teacher and financial analyst combined with specialized studies allowed him to broaden his academic vision and include practical analysis for making investment decisions, whether evaluating productive projects or financial investments.

He is passionate about writing because he believes that it is a way to share knowledge and experiences with the rest of the world, he hopes to contribute concepts and ideas that improve people's quality of life, both materially and personally.

INTRODUCTION

During the years I studied economics I had to constantly face critics and comments about how useless my career was in real life, the overconsumption of assumptions in the theories and models we studied. Many others claimed that it was almost impossible to find a good job as an economist unless it was in politics, teaching, or research and that he better studies some engineering or something else ""applied"." Today, after some time of my studies I can say that these people are largely right, the economy they teach in most universities around the world is based more on the understanding of complex models that are inconsistent with reality than in the study of the world economy, its evolution, its evolution and the understanding of its dynamics. In my opinion, this is mainly due to the "balance" paradigm, we are dedicated to studying the necessary conditions for a so-called market to find balance through the law of supply and demand, to identify what are the possible failures in the process and to propose regulations so that these failures do not occur, and reach the point of "efficiency". And is that the market is not a place where buyers and sellers are to buy or sell a product, the market is a dynamic and evolutionary environment that is part of the daily life of all the forgiveness that inhabits this planet, has naturally emerged from the interaction between people and allowed us to improve the living conditions of most of us, pretending to find a balance point where all the products of the economy were bought and sold at certain prices, is to try to freeze the time to find a "solution" that would possibly be useless for the next minute after having "found" it.

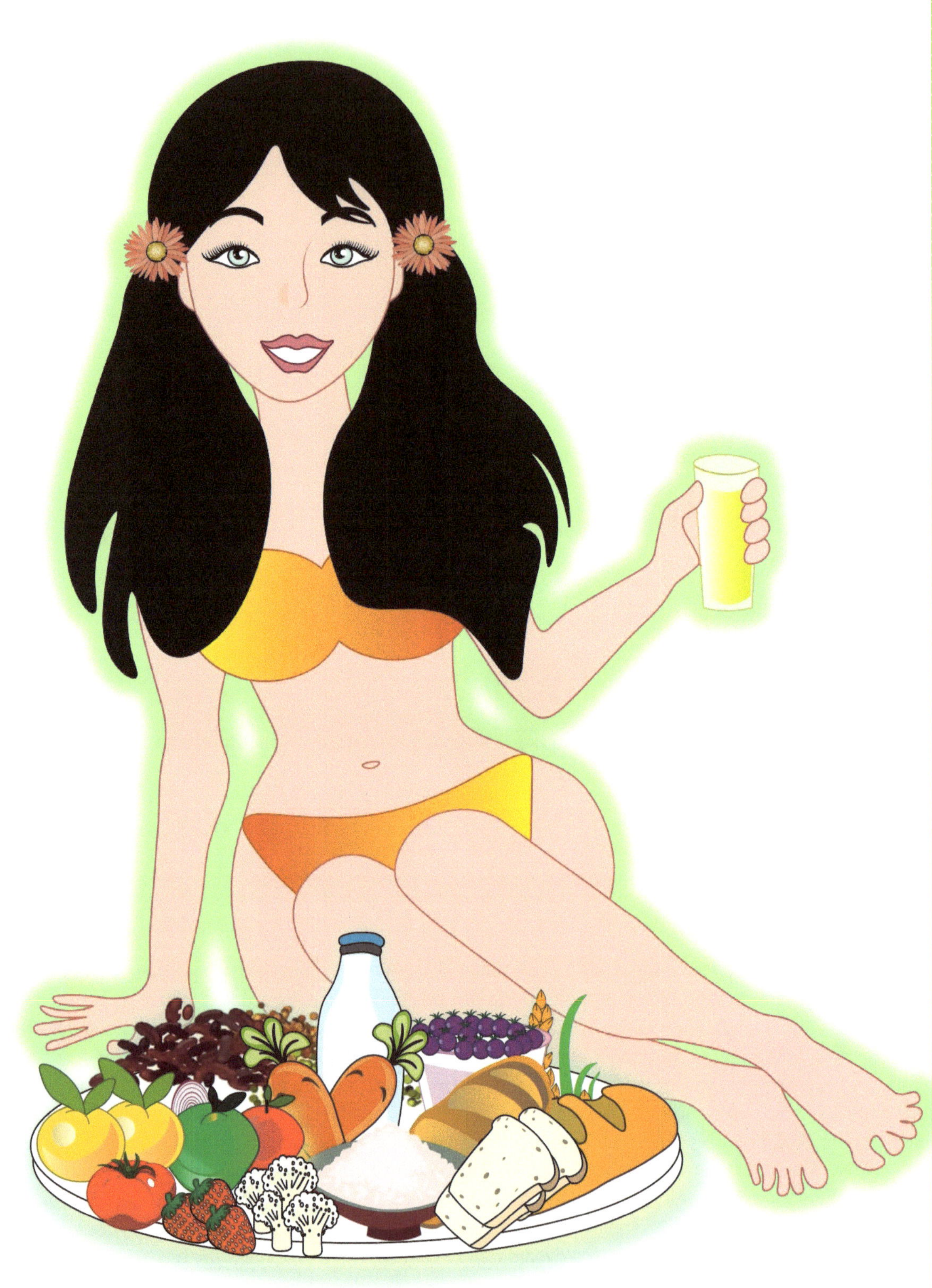

NOMBRE	CARACTERISTICA	CANTIDAD	ALIMENTOS QUE LO CONTIENEN
VITAMINA A (Retinol, Retinal, ácido Retinoico)	Importante para el crecimiento y desarrollo. Para el mantenimiento del sistema inmunológico y para una buena visión.	800 Mcg o 0,0008 Gramos	Aceite de Hígado de bacalao. Hígado de pavo, res, cerdo, pescado o pollo. Ghee. Batata, zanahoria, hoja de brócoli. Mantequilla, col rizada, calabaza. Diente de león, espinaca, queso chédar, melón, pimiento, huevo, albaricoque, papaya, tomate, mango, guisante, leche, espirulina. Ternera.

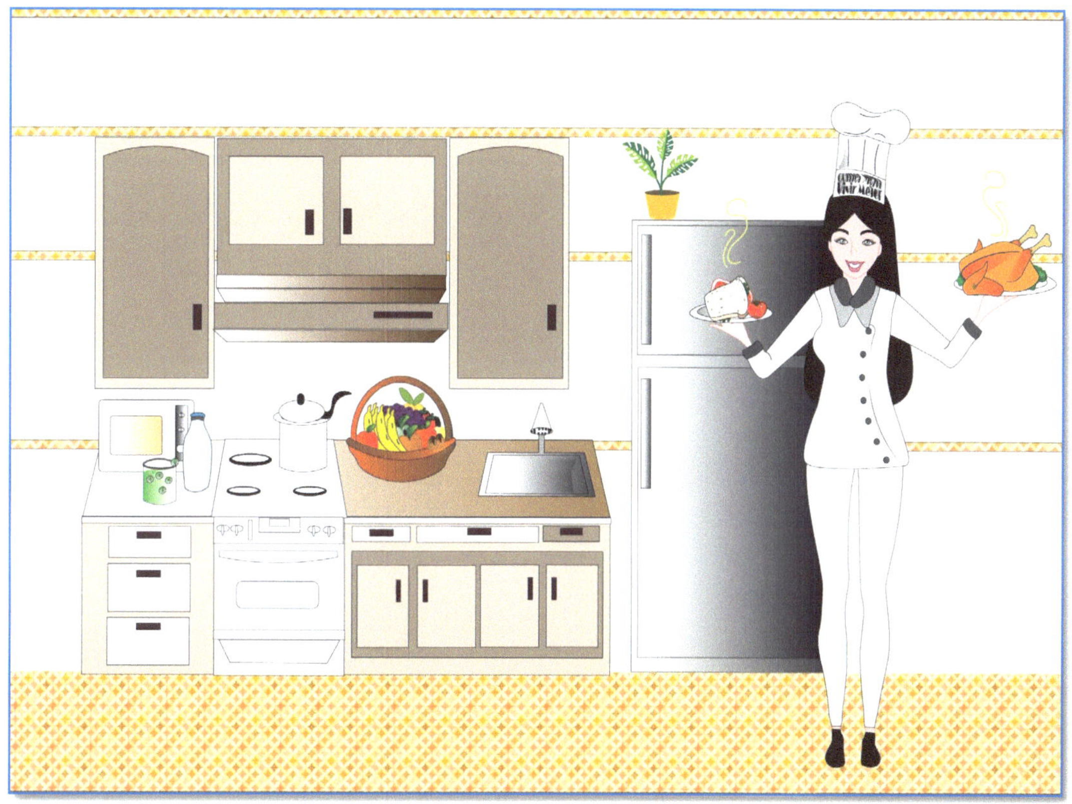

Nutrition is a biological process through which organisms assimilate the food and fluids necessary for movement, growth and maintenance of their vital functions. Nutrition also has to do with the relationship between food and health and especially in determining a balanced diet based on the Food Pyramid.

Good nutrition considers the processes of absorption, digestion, metabolism and excretion. It also considers the correct combination of foods and the anti-nutritional factors of some of those foods you eat.

DEFINE NUTRITION

But Nutrition is not based only on some concepts, nutrition is also about the way we eat, that everything we eat must be balanced and that balance must be specifically focused on the metabolism of each being. human.

Remember that all human beings are different and that in the process of nutrition these differences are very marked.

Generalizing nutrition without considering the way in which each person absorbs the nutrients from their food, the way they metabolize them and the way they expel them from their body, whether they expel them or not, is perhaps one of the biggest mistakes some nutritionists make.

Each person has different needs in all aspects of his life, especially in nutrition.

But what is metabolism? It is the ability of living beings to chemically change the nature of the substances they consume through chemical reactions and physicochemical processes that occur in cells and the body. And that capacity is totally individual. Therein lies the importance of taking the Nutrition process individually, wondering, investigating, taking the time to realize how food works in your own body. God made us perfect, your body talks to you, your body tells you when food is good or bad for you.

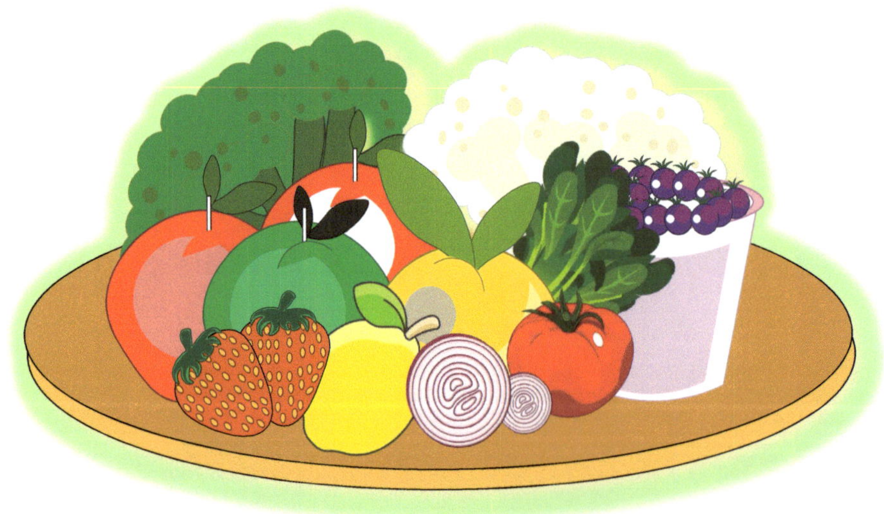

DEFINE NUTRITION

With good nutrition we achieve a notable and progressive increase in energy and a decrease in digestive problems. We will improve our physical appearance and rejuvenate ourselves inside and out.

We also strengthen the immune system systematically. We have an easier time losing weight without starving. We increase the joviality and mental clarity.

Being well nourished we can overcome all the physical demands of our day to day. We stay awake, attentive and focused on the perfect performance of our tasks, both personally and professionally. We will be more efficient in our work and we will overcome all the obstacles that come our way every day.

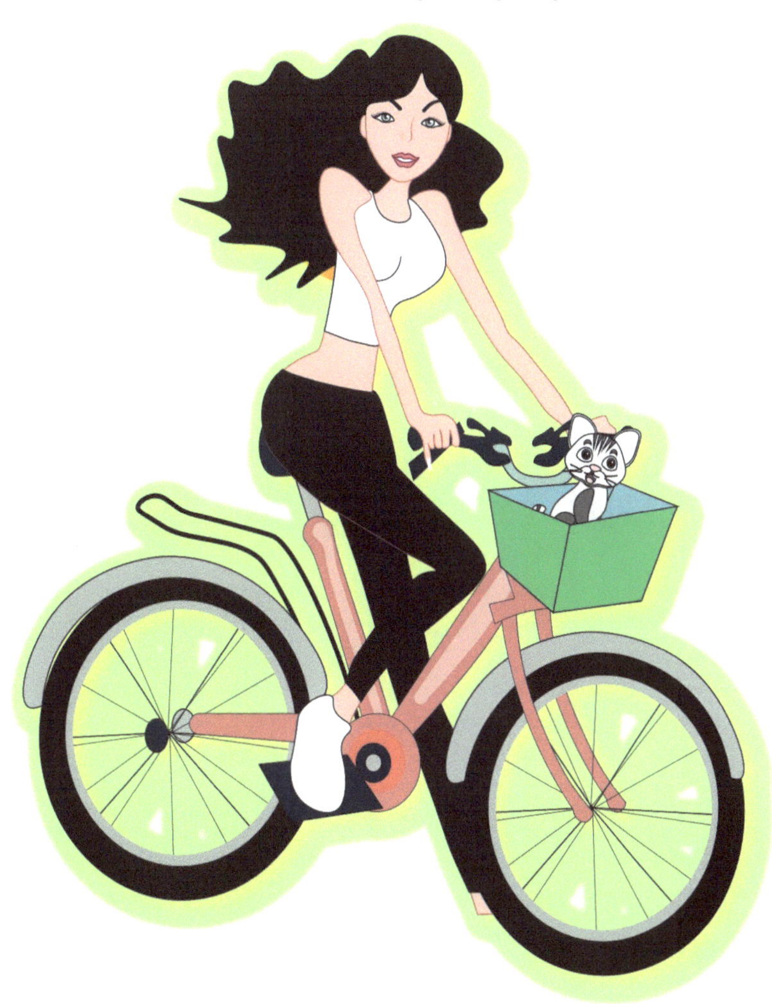

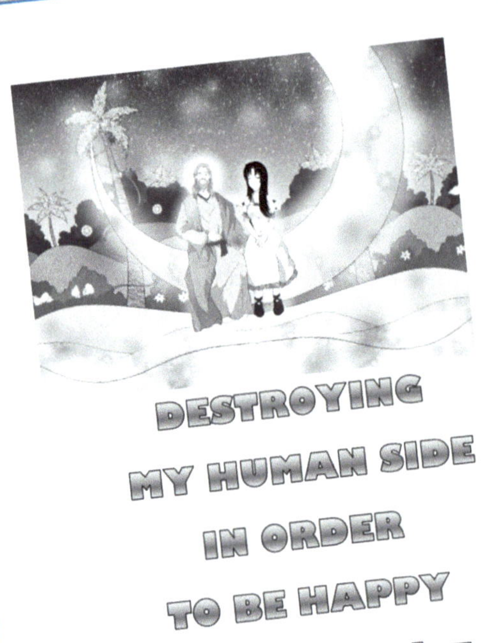

DESTROYING MY HUMAN SIDE IN ORDER TO BE HAPPY

Gladys Méndez

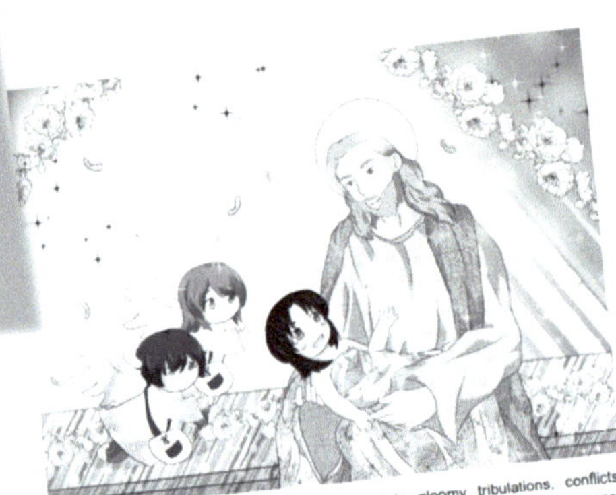

In the complete darkness of a universe lost in gloomy tribulations, conflicts, disappointments and heartbreakes, the light of hope is reborn with the divine presence of God, within the heart of every human being.

It was the month of July of the year one thousand nine hundred and sixty-four. Year of great world events. Wars, chaos and destruction roamed the earth and unbelief seized humanity.

But during that chaos, there in heaven, in that world of peace, where the wonderful is possible, where the alpha and the omega come from and where happiness always reigns, standing on a white cloud, was God speaking with the Angel Miguel. He asked her to go to the secret crypt to tell Angel Joel to prepare the dones of the baby Johan, because she was the only one missing to receive them and she was among the group of those who would travel to earth the next day.

The Angel Miguel obeyed the orders of the Lord, walked through the clouds crossing the sky from east to west, he gets to the tree of absolute truth, covered by white flowers and green leaves, all equal in size and shape, raised his right arm, he made a circular gesture of reverence with his hand and the tree opened its stem to make way for the main entrance of the crypt.

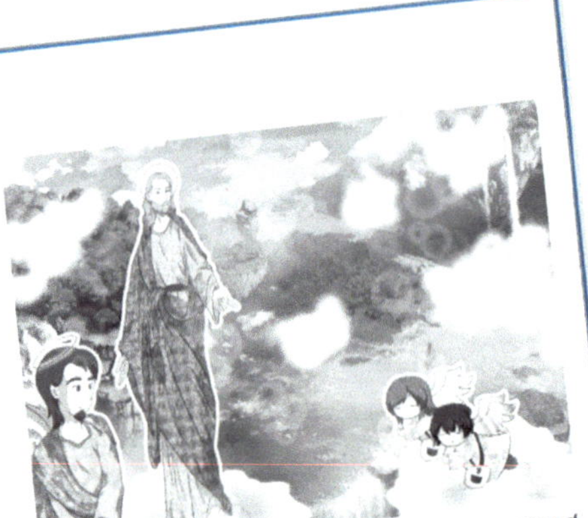

He found the Angel Joel mixing the elixir consecrated with fine oils and essences of exquisite aromas that permeated the room and traveled through the environment enveloping everything. He transmitted the message of the Lord, warned him to follow the instructions to the letter to prevent him from making a mistake and left. The Angel Joel waited until The Angel Miguel retreated to approach the window of his laboratory and observe from a distance, the smiling face of baby Johan, who was sleeping peacefully on a hammock, with guardian angels around her, in charge of watching over her dream.

The baby, looked so tender, that the Angel Joel decided to ignore the warnings of Angel Miguel and created for her an extra portion of the gift of sensitivity that he put in a tiny glass cylinder along with the other gifts, faith, hope, love, forgiveness, wisdom, patience, understanding, piety and fear of God. Then he went in search of the baby Johan to provide her with the gifts that would mark his destiny forever. Just when Angel Joel finished his mission and since all the creatures were ready to leave, the clouds darkened, the firmament was dyed red, the sky was filled with resplendent stars that directed the flash of its light towards the babies and they unloaded on them all the power of their luminosity. Then they went out, leaving the sky in complete darkness.

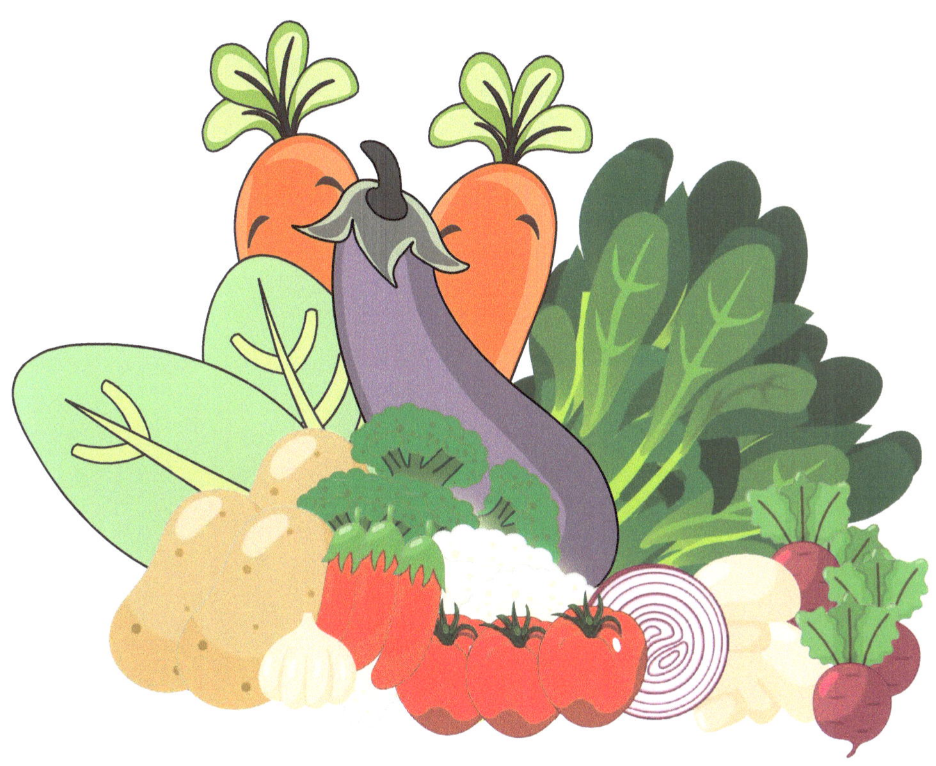

Three-quarters of the food we consume must be alkaline, which are those rich in minerals, such as fruits and vegetables. The other quarter must be acidic, especially proteins.

Do not consume excess calories, have a low-fat diet, eat a variety of foods, reduce salt intake, limit the consumption of cured, smoked, baked and fried foods. Consume sugar in moderation. Respect the four meals, breakfast, lunch, snack and dinner.

NUTRITIONAL DEMANDS

We must consume 4 to 6 servings a day of cereals, they are a source of fiber and vitamins. It is recommended to eat them whole.

We must consume two units a day of dairy products, since they are a source of calcium and vitamins A, D and E, they are of high nutritional value. They are antioxidants.

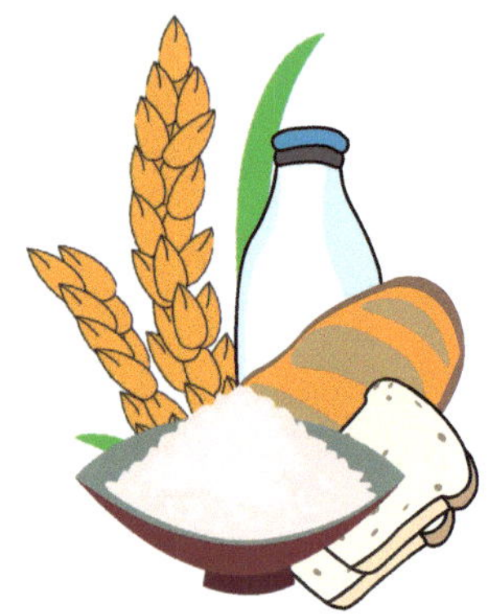

We must consume at least one or two servings a day of vegetables and greens. They do not have cholesterol, They are rich in healthy fibers composed of carbohydrates, polysaccharides, proteins and healthy fats and have low caloric density.

We must consume at least 4 fruits a day, the fruits provide fiber, vitamins, minerals, antioxidants, flavonoids, soil, selenium and have a high-water content of 80 to 95%. Fruits are an inexhaustible source of healthy compounds for our body, easily absorbed and digested. It is recommended to eat them alone to get the most out of them.

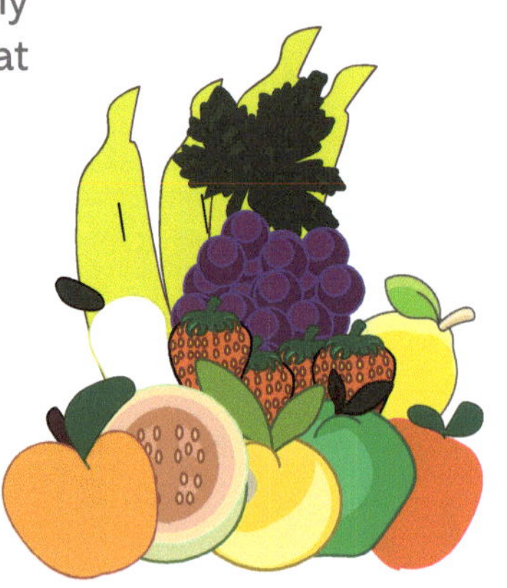

Of the dairy products, yogurt stands out since its fats are better digested and contain probiotics that have a beneficial effect on our intestinal health.

As for cheeses, for people who suffer from hypertension, it is recommended to eat skimmed cheeses as they are lower in salt.

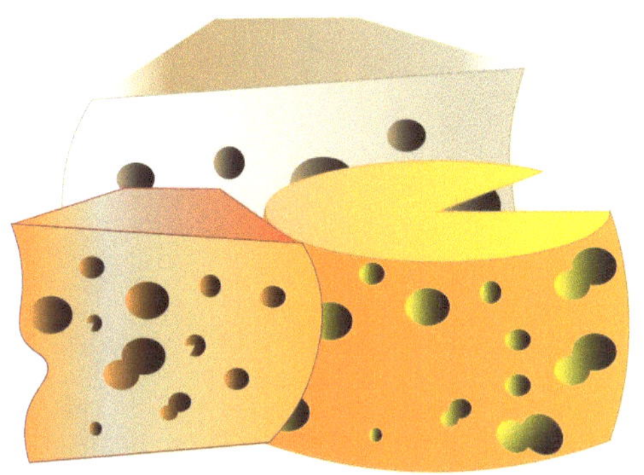

We must consume 30 to 60 grams a day of fats and oils, they are high in calories and energy, being fats of animal origin the ones that are richer in saturated fatty acids.

We must consume 3 to 7 weekly servings of nuts since they contain easily absorbed minerals, they contain vitamins A, B1, iron, calcium. Walnuts are specifically better for the heart.

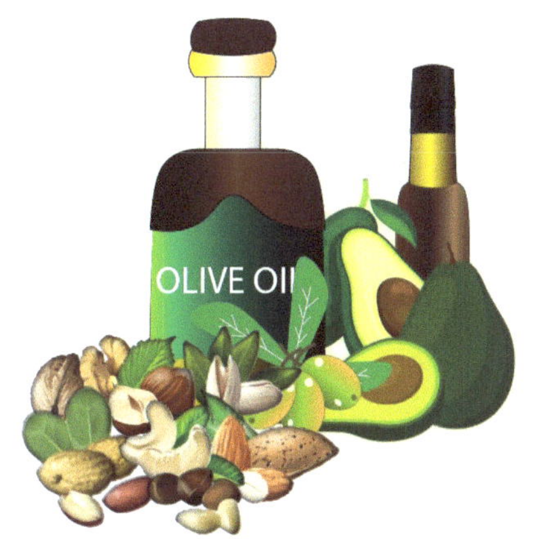

We must consume 3 to 4 weekly servings of fish as they provide 18% of proteins of biological value, they are a source of B vitamins, especially B1 and B2.

They provide vitamins A and D, they are rich in iodine, phosphorus, potassium, magnesium and calcium. They contribute to digestibility and are the best sources of omega 3 acids.

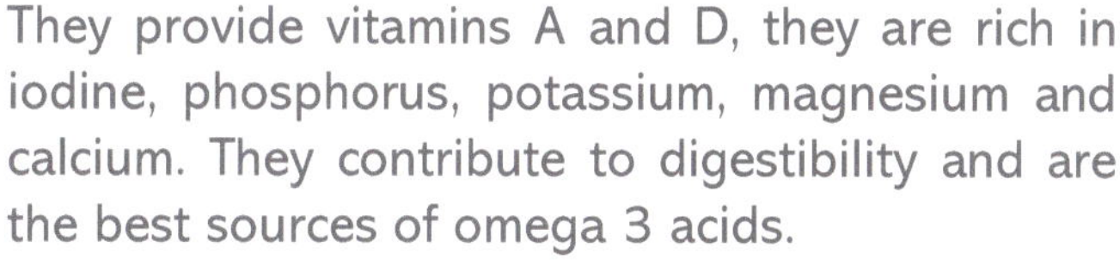
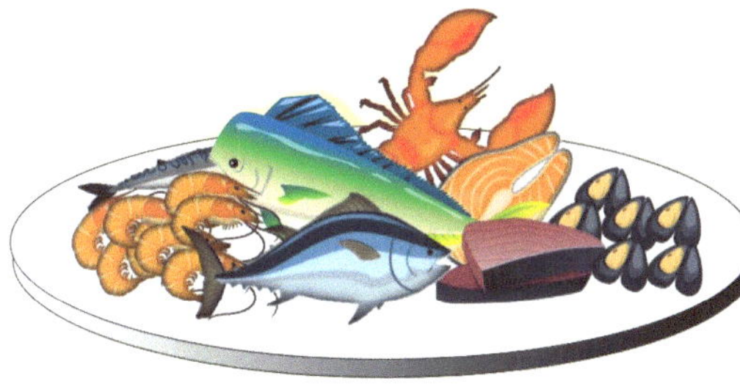

We must consume 3 to 5 eggs a week, they are a source of many vitamins and minerals and have very good quality proteins of high biological value. It is recommended to cook the egg well.

NUTRITIONAL DEMANDS

We must consume 3 to 4 weekly servings of meat, since they are a good source of vitamins, especially those of group B, they provide proteins of high biological value and contain all the essential amino acids

They are rich in iron, provide minerals, zinc, potassium and phosphorus. Except for the visors that are poor in vitamins A, C, folic acid, and carbohydrates.

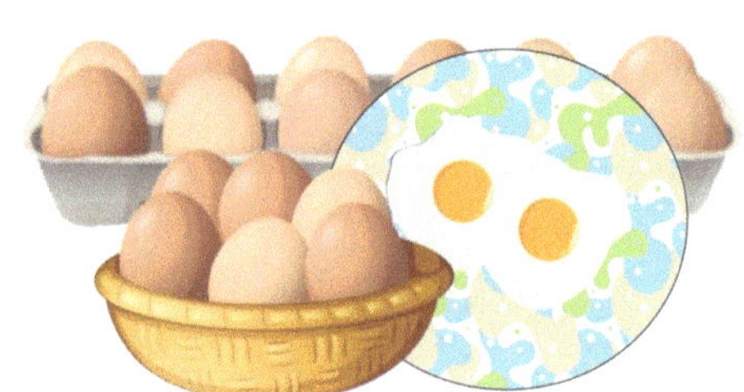

It is advisable to remove the fat and the skin, cook on the grill, boiled, roast, grill and not fry them. Do not eat cold cuts.

Finally, it is advisable to season meals with spices such as turmeric, saffron, cinnamon and pepper, since they stimulate the secretion of gastric juices, increase the digestibility of some foods, contribute to good blood pressure, have antimicrobial properties, vitamins A and C and lots of antioxidants and polyphenols.

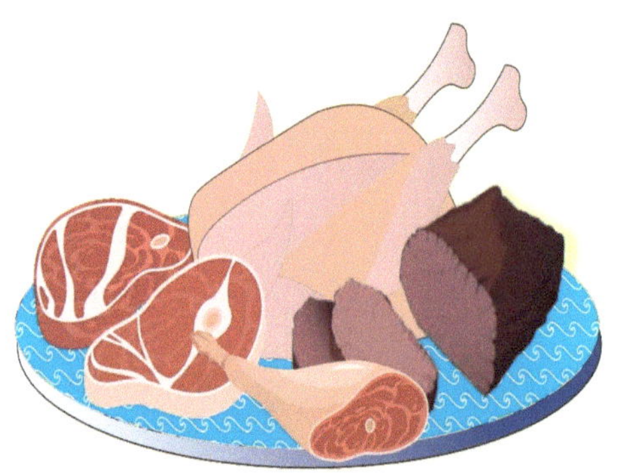

All legumes, except lentils and peas, must be soaked the night before they are prepared and when cooking three parts of water to one part of legumes must be used.

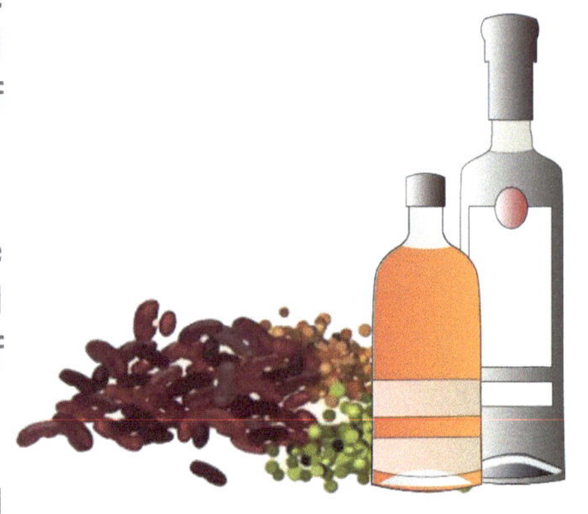

Let it boil for 10 minutes over rapid heat and uncovered to remove the foam that appears on top and add the salt at the end of cooking. (Be careful to put next to the legumes).

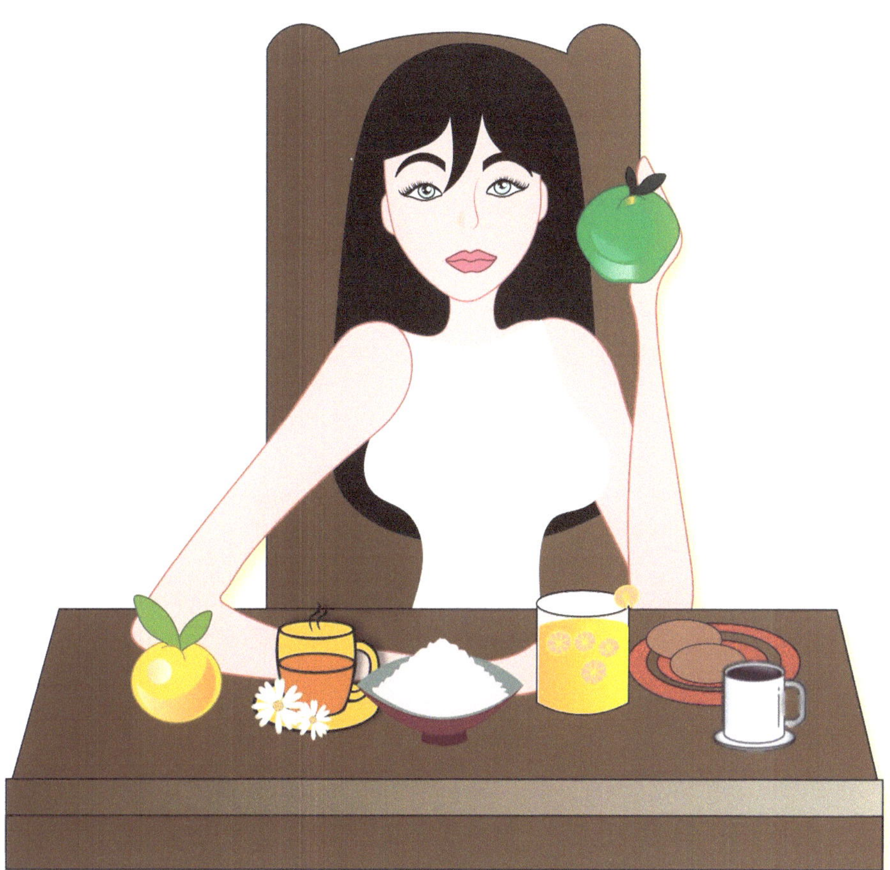

The digestive process begins in the mouth, which, together with the teeth, the tongue and the salivary glands, convert the food we eat into the bolus that is then transported through the pharynx, passes through the esophagus and then reaches the stomach where it is accumulate food.

Once in the stomach, hydrochloric acid breaks down food proteins and some fats, but to a lesser extent. The food mixes with the gastric juices and the mucus produced by the secretory glands of the stomach, forming a semi-liquid substance called chyme which has been transferred to the small intestine to continue digestion.

THE DIGESTION

The pancreas and liver also generate juices and substances that pass into the small intestine to bind with the chyme to continue the digestive process.

The small intestine is responsible for absorbing nutrients from already digested food to take them to the blood. Then the food that was not absorbed passes to the large intestine that takes it to the anus to be discarded.

For human beings to have a good digestion, it is necessary to consider the time in which food remains in the stomach before passing to the small intestine.

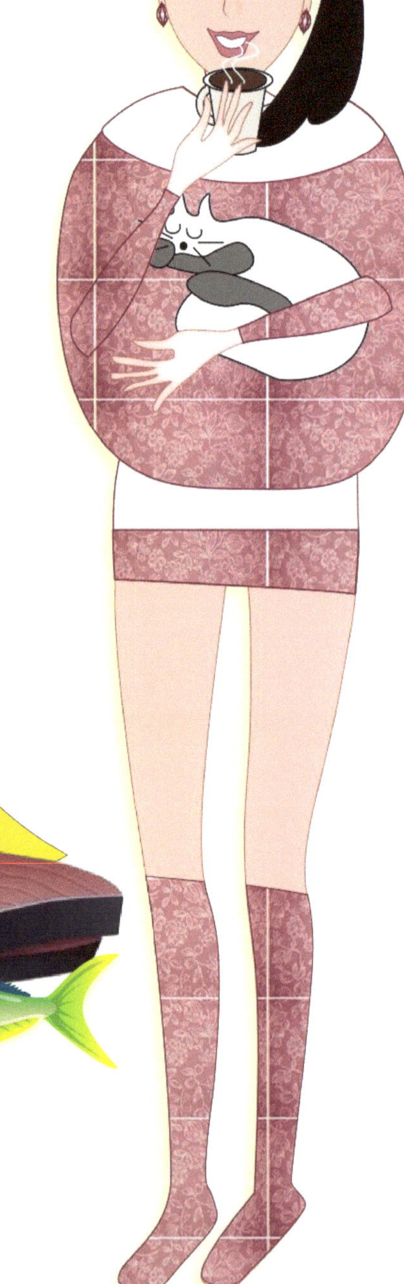

There are many ways to keep our immune system strong, external elements and internal elements.

Some examples of external elements:

Try to reduce stress through relaxation, meditation, breathing exercises, yoga, and martial arts such as Tai Chi.

Being in constant contact with nature and exercising. Walk for at least 20 minutes a day.

STRENGTHENING THE IMMUNE SYSTEM

Get enough sleep each day. Take vitamin C to increase the production of cells that fight infection.

Eat healthy. Include probiotics in the daily diet and drink enough water, 10 to 12 glasses of 250 milliliters.

Don't smoke, try to maintain a healthy weight, don't drink alcohol, or drink in moderation.

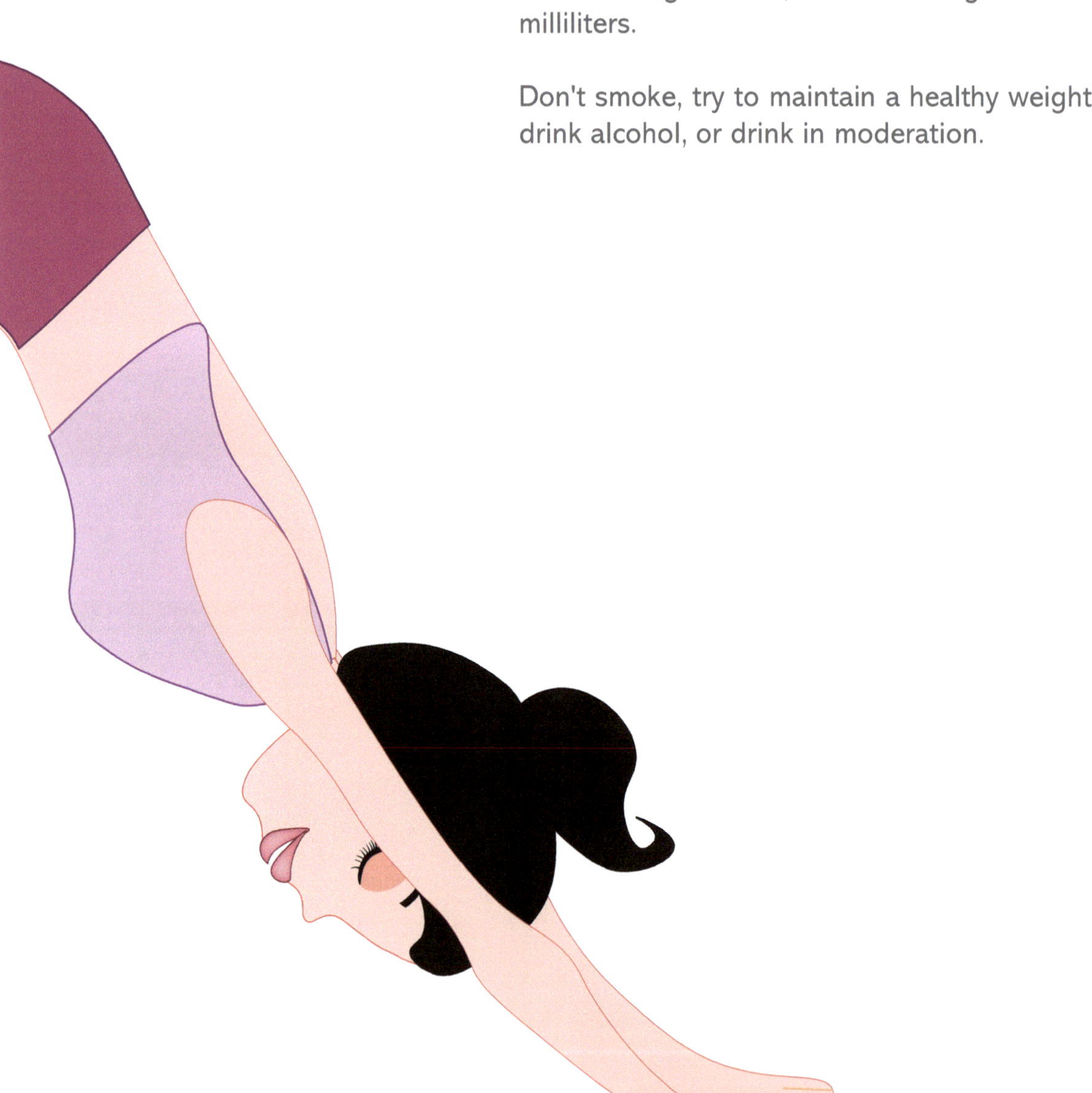

FOOD PROPERTIES

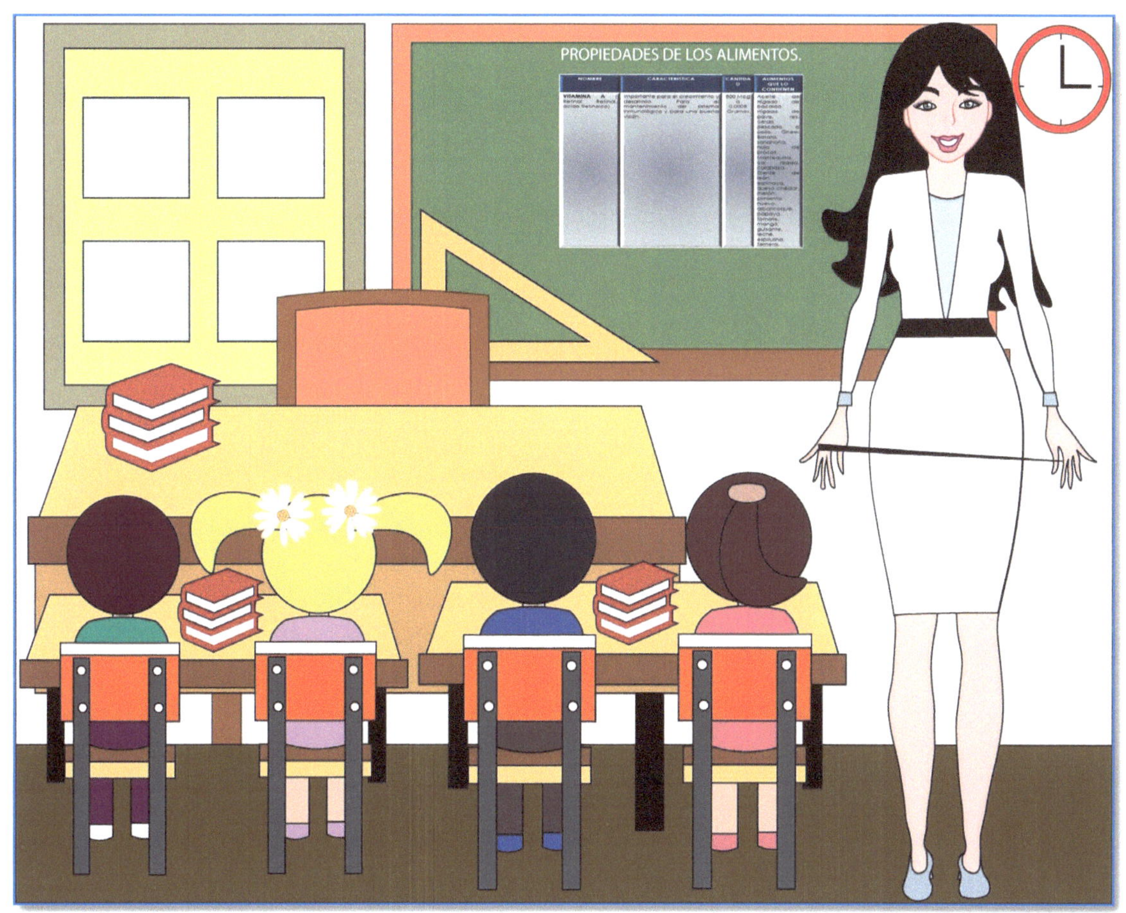

Food is substances that are incorporated into the body and are transformed into cells and body secretions. Foods are classified into proteins, carbohydrates (which are sugars and starches), fruits, fats, vegetables, and greens.

All foods contain vitamins, proteins and minerals that are absorbed by the body and constitute nutrition.

Here's a list of some of the vitamins, proteins, and minerals, the daily amount needed for good nutrition, and the foods that contain them.

FOOD PROPERTIES

NAME	CHARACTERISTIC	QUANTITY	FOODS THAT CONTAIN IT
VITAMIN A (Retinol, Retinal, Retinoic acid)	Important for growth and development. For the maintenance of the immune system and for good vision.	800 Mcg or 0.0008 Grams	Cod Liver Oil. Turkey, beef, pork, fish, or chicken liver. Ghee. Sweet potato, carrot, broccoli leaf. Butter, kale, pumpkin. Dandelion, spinach, cheddar cheese, melon, pepper, egg, apricot, papaya, tomato, mango, pea, milk, spirulina. Veal.

NAME	CHARACTERISTIC	QUANTITY	FOODS THAT CONTAIN IT
VITAMIN B1 (Thiamine)	It helps convert all the food we eat into energy. Important for the growth and development of the body's cells.	1, 2 Miligrams	Yeast, wheat germ, bread, pasta, legumes, whole grains. Oats, wheat, corn, nuts. Eggs, visors, pork, beef, liver, fish. Potatoes.

NAME	CHARACTERISTIC	QUANTITY	FOODS THE CONTAIN IT
VITAMIN B2 (Riboflavin)	It has an important role in energy metabolism. It is necessary for the integrity of the skin, mucosa, and cornea. Detoxifies the body of harmful substances. Participates in the metabolism of other vitamins.	1,4 Miligrams	Meats, dairy, cereals, yeast and green vegetables. Liver, dried herbs, spices and peppers. Almonds, edamame, bran, wheat germ. Fish, salmon, sesame seeds. Dry tomatoes.

NAME	CHARACTERISTIC	QUANTITY	FOODS THAT CONTAIN IT
VITAMIN B3 (Niacin, nicotinic acid, vitamin PP)	Elimination of toxic chemicals in the body, participates in the production of steroid hormones, powerful rubefacient. Indispensable to use the metabolic energy of food. Fundamental for growth. Keeps the nervous and circulatory system in good condition. Maintains healthy skin, stabilizes blood glucose, and restores DNA.	16 Miligrams	Palm hearts, mushrooms, garlic, asparagus, banana, propolis, broccoli, carrot, sweet potatoes, yeast extract, wheat bran, rice, fish, anchovies, tuna, swordfish. Liver, paprika, peanuts, beef, chicken, bacon, sun-dried tomatoes, vegetables.

NAME	CHARACTERISTIC	QUANTITY	FOODS THAT CONTAIN IT
VITAMIN B5 (Pantothenic acid)	It is an essential factor for many of the chemical reactions that occur in our body and that are necessary for the proper functioning of the human body.	6 Miligrams	Liver, kidneys, bran, sunflower seed, whey powder, egg yolk, tomatoes, cheese, fish, avocado.

NAME	CHARACTERISTIC	QUANTITY	FOODS THAT CONTAIN IT
VITAMIN B6 (Pyridoxine)	It is essential for the functioning of the enzymes that are the proteins that regulate the chemical processes of the body.	1,4 Miligrams	Wheat germ, meat, eggs, fish, vegetables, legumes, nuts, enriched breads and cereals. Chicken, turkey, beef, pork, fish, cod, salmon, trout, tuna. Spinach, broccoli.

FOOD PROPERTIES

NAME	CHARACTERISTIC	QUANTITY	FOODS THAT CONTAIN IT
VITAMIN B8 (Vitamin H, vitamin 7)	Essential for the synthesis and degradation of fats and certain amino acids.	50 Micro grams o 0,005 Grms	Liver, dairy products, vegetables, eggs, fish, legumes, whole grains, yeast. Lentil, chickpea, beans, soybeans, vegetables, peanuts, peas, walnuts, rice, milk, fruits.

NAME	CHARACTERISTIC	QUANTITY	FOODS THAT CONTAIN IT
VITAMIN B9 (Folic Acid)	Helps in tissue growth and cell work. Helps the body break down, use, and create new proteins.	200 Micro grams or 0,0002 Grms	Spinach, Cabbage, Lettuce, Milk, Fruits, Vegetables, Eggs, Meat, Nuts.

NAME	CHARACTERISTIC	QUANTITY	FOODS THAT CONTAIN IT
VITAMIN B12 (Cobalamin)	Ideal for the normal functioning of the brain, the nervous system, for the formation of blood and various proteins. Involved in the metabolism of the cells of the human body, especially DNA. It also contributes to the metabolization of amino acids, fatty acids and carbohydrates.	2,5 Micro grams 0,000025 Grms	Beef liver, clams, fish, shellfish, meat, poultry, eggs, milk. Yeast, cereals.

FOOD PROPERTIES

NAME	CHARACTERISTIC	QUANTITY	FOODS THAT CONTAIN IT
VITAMIN C	It is a powerful antioxidant that has beneficial effects on the immune system and the aging process, endothelial integrity and lipoprotein metabolism. Prevents premature aging, facilitates the absorption of other vitamins and minerals. It prevents degenerative diseases and heart disease, helps collagen production.	8 Miligrams	Fruits and vegetables, guavas, red pepper, parsley, kiwi, grape, Brussels sprouts, papaya, strawberry, orange, lemon, melon, cauliflower, pineapple, mint, grapefruit, raspberry, mandarin, spinach, raw cabbage, mango, lime.

NAME	CHARACTERISTIC	QUANTITY	FOODS THAT CONTAIN IT
VITAMIN D	Essential substance for calcium metabolism and bone mineralization. Regulates calcium and phosphate levels at the renal level. It contributes to bone formation, indispensable for the proper functioning of the human skeleton.	5 Micro grams	Cod liver oil, tuna, salmon, mackerel and sardine. Beef liver and egg yolk. Mushrooms and mushrooms. The sun's rays.

NAME	CHARACTERISTIC	QUANTITY	FOODS THAT CONTAIN IT
VITAMIN K	It is involved in blood clotting. It has a protective effect against liver cancer, leukemia, lung, colon, oral, breast and bladder cancer.	75 Micro grams	Cabbage, spinach, turnips, mustard leaves, parsley, lettuce, broccoli, cauliflower.

FOOD PROPERTIES

NAME	CHARACTERISTIC	QUANTITY	FOODS THAT CONTAIN IT
VITAMIN E	It has a fundamental role in the normal metabolism of cells. It is the most important fat-soluble antioxidant in human and animal tissues. Protects fatty acids against oxidative damage.	12 Miligrams	Broccoli, spinach, soybeans. Brewer's yeast, egg yolk. Vegetable oils, nuts, almonds. Margarine.

NAME	CHARACTERISTIC	QUANTITY	FOODS THAT CONTAIN IT
POTASSIUM	It is involved in normal water balance, osmotic balance and muscle contraction and the regulation of neuromuscular activity.	2000 Miligrams	Potato, cauliflower, broccoli, beet, eggplant.

NAME	CHARACTERISTIC	QUANTITY	FOODS THAT CONTAIN IT
CHLORINE	It favors proper blood circulation, helps prevent heart attacks, stabilizes blood pressure, relieves bronchitis, promotes good digestion, prevents kidney stones, improves the immune system.	800 Miligrams	Bulgur, sea salt, barley, cooked spinach, pumpkin seeds, cornmeal, black beans, roasted almonds.

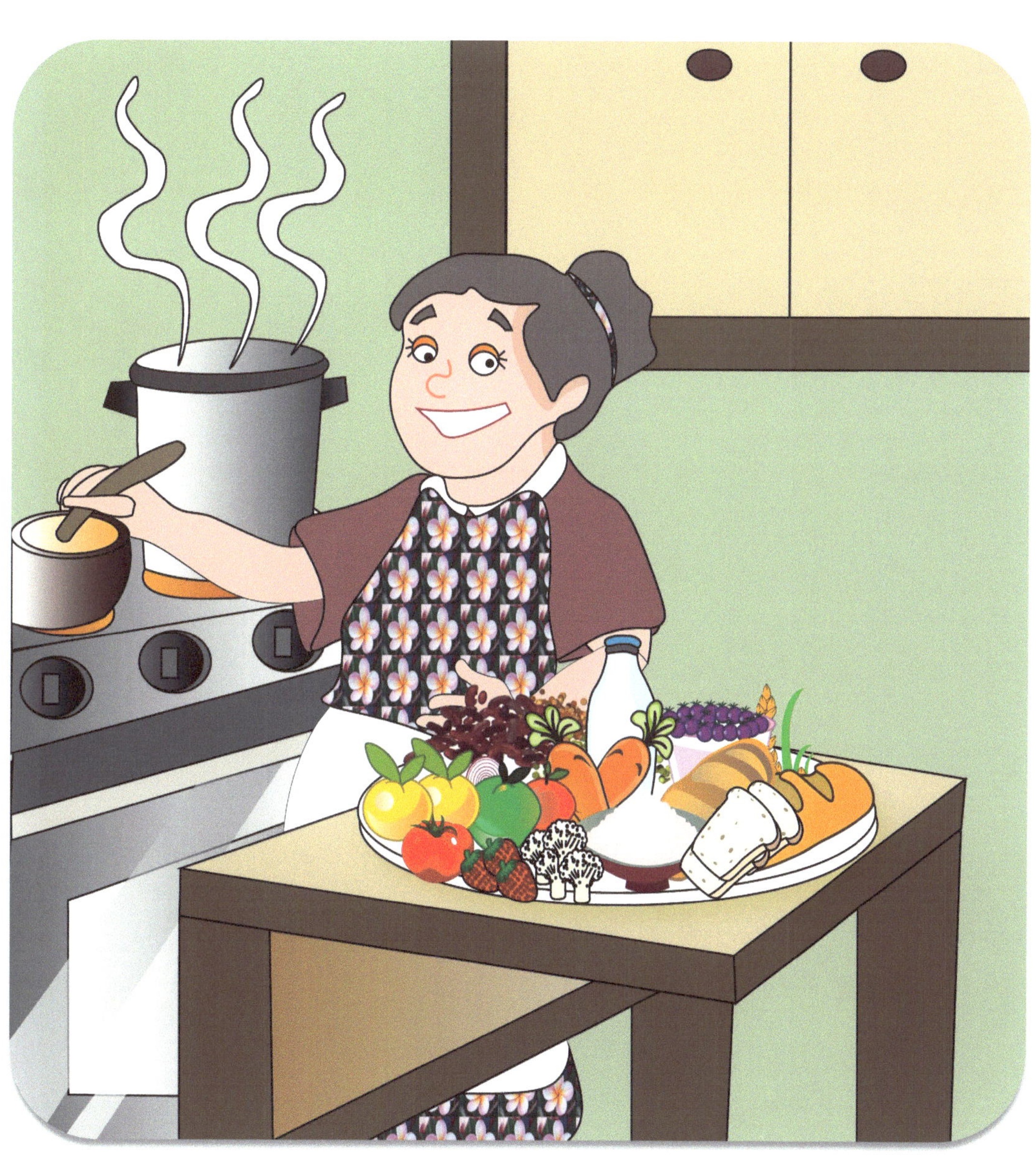

HEALTHY SALADS

CUCUMBER, TOMATO AND AVOCADO

INGREDIENTS:

2 CUCUMBERS
6 CHERRY TOMATOES
¼ OF MOZZARELA CHEESE
½ AVOCADO
½ RED ONION
1 TBSP APPLE VINEGAR
½ LEMON
1 PINCH OF SALT

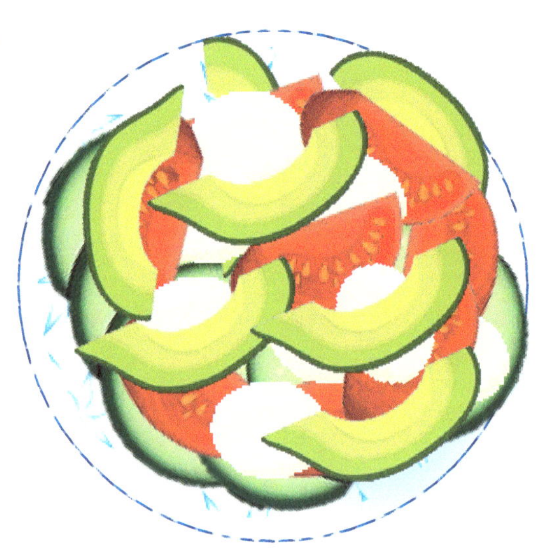

SPINACH AND POTATO

INGREDIENTS:

4 COOKED POTATOES
1/2 POUND FINELY
CHOPPED SPINACH
2 WARM EGGS
A PINCH OF SALT

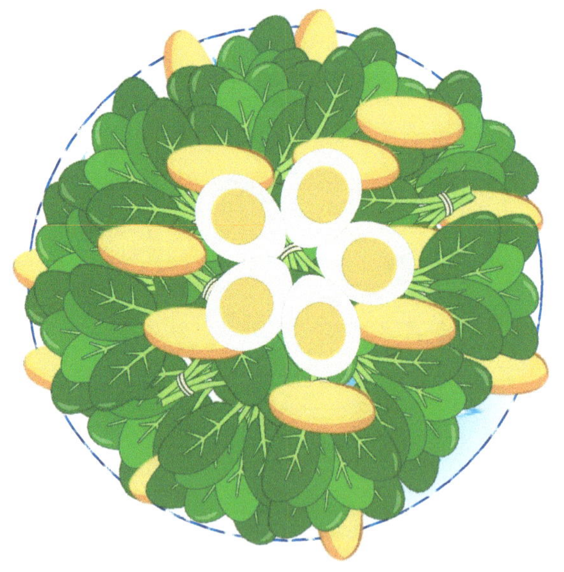

HEALTHY SALADS

CELERY, OLIVES, WHOLE-GRAIN CROQUETTES

INGREDIENTS:

3 CELERY BRANCHES
10 BLACK OLIVES, WHOLE OR
CUT INTO PIECES
2 TOMATOES
Toast
1 GREEN PEPPER
1 LEMON
COME TO TASTE

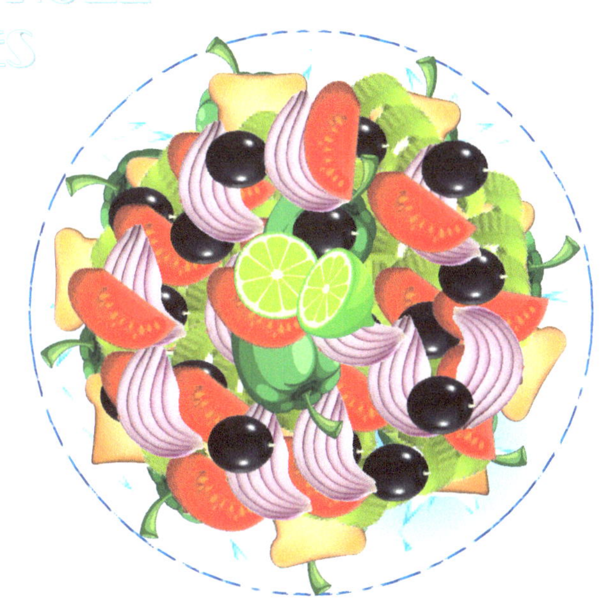

SPINACH, COMMAND AND RED CRANBERRIES

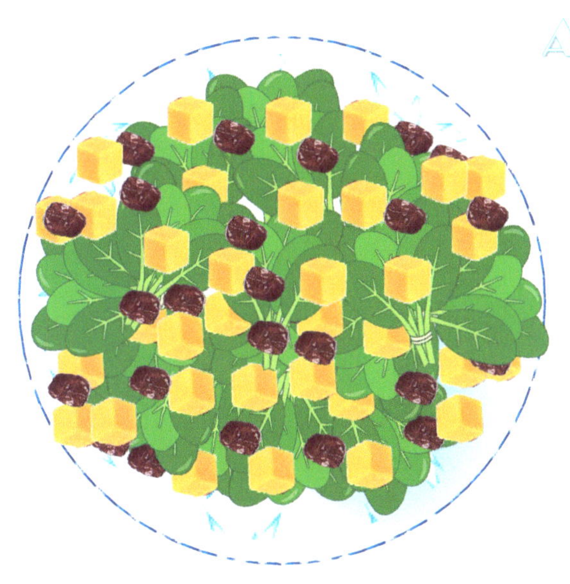

INGREDIENTS:

1/2 POUND SPINACH
1 RIPE MANGO CUT
INTO SQUARES
1/2 POUND DRIED
CRANBERRIES
OLIVE OIL
1/2 LEMON
1 PINCH OF SALT

HEALTHY SALADS

BEETS, CARROTS AND POTATOES

INGREDIENTS:

3 COOKED BEETS AND SPLIT
INTO SMALL PIECES
2 CARROTS COOKED IN
SLICES
2 SLICED COOKED POTATOES
1 RED-EGG ONION IN
JULIENNE
1,/ LIMON
COME TO TASTE
CHOPPED CORIANDER FOR
GARNISH

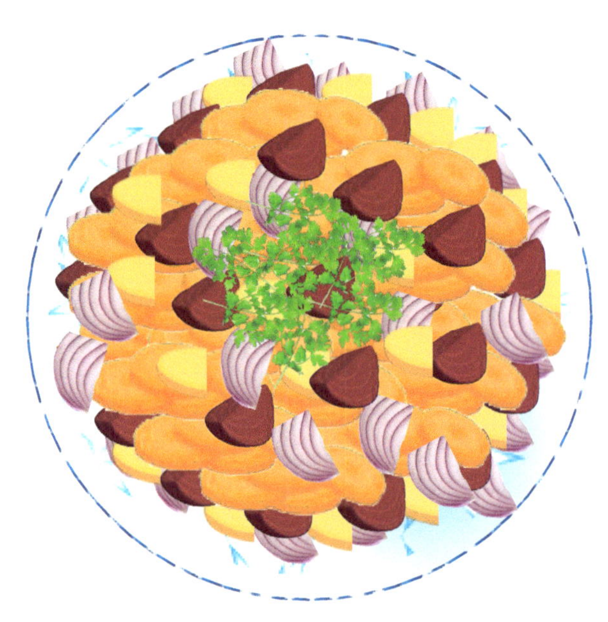

BROCCOLI, CARROT AND NUTS

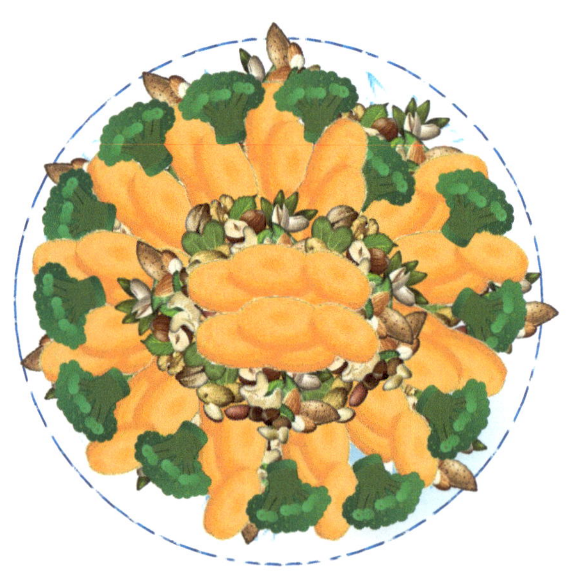

INGREDIENTS:

1 BUNCH OF BROCCOLI
2 CARROTS
ALMONDS AND WALNUTS
1 TABLESPOON OLIVE OIL
1 TABLESPOON APPLE CIDER
COME TO TASTE

HEALTHY SALADS

TUNA, POTATO AND CELERY

INGREDIENTES:

1 CAN OF TUNA IN
WATER
3 COOKED POTATOES
1/2 RED EGG ONION
2 RED PEPPERS
2 CELERY STALKS, CUT
INTO SQUARES
CILANTRO FOR GARNISH
1/2 LEMON
COME TO TASTE

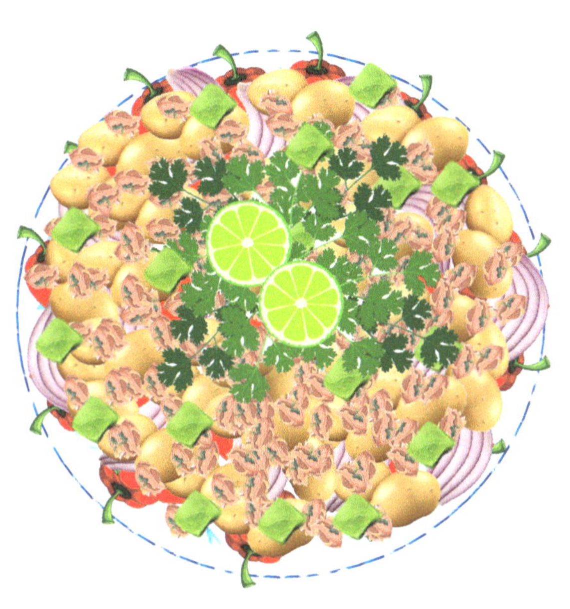

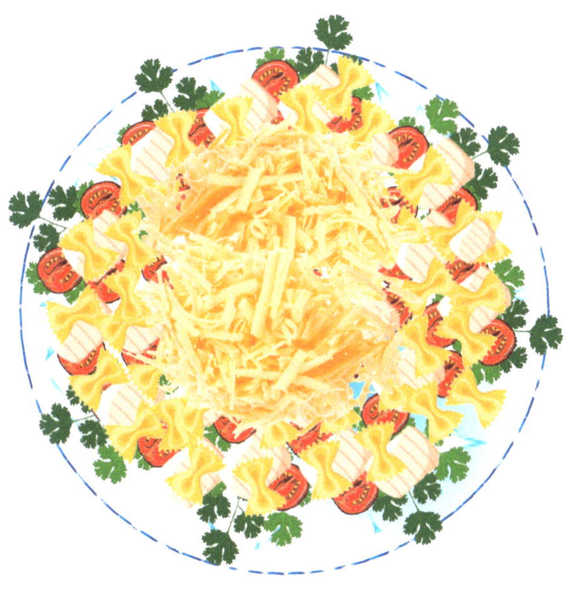

PASTA, CHICKEN AND TOMATO

INGREDIENTS:

1/2 POUND COOKED PASTA
CILANTRO BRANCHES
HALF A POUND OF CHERRY
TOMATO
HALF A POUND OF FINELY
CHOPPED ROAST CHICKEN
PARMESAN CHEESE TO
TASTE

HEALTHY SALADS

AVOCADO AND ONION

INGREDIENTS:

1 AVOCADO CUT IN JULIENNED
1 RED EGG ONION
1 RIPE MANGO CUT INTO
SQUARES
MOZZARELA CHEESE
1 TABLESPOON OLIVE OIL
1/2 LEMON
COME TO TASTE

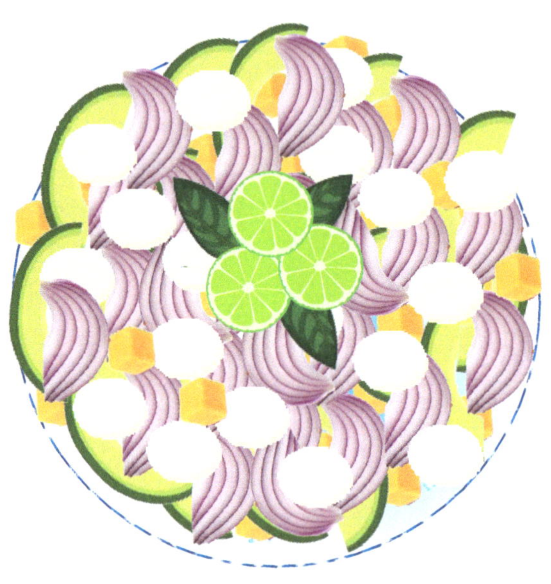

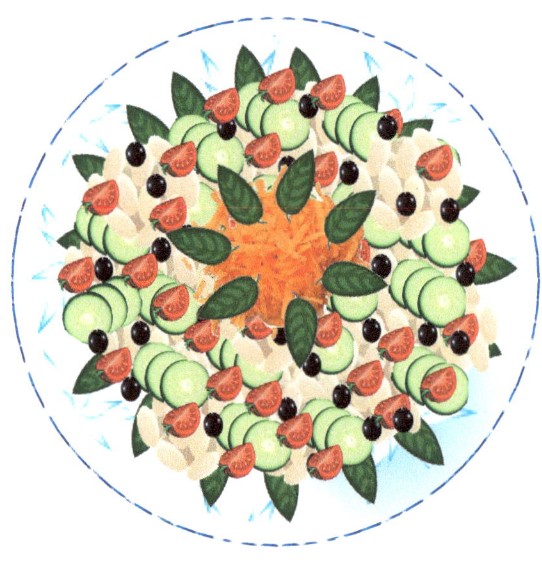

RICE, TOMATO AND CUCUMBER

INGREDIENTS:

1/2 POUND RICE
1 CUCUMBER, SLICED
1 TOMATO, FINELY CHOPPED
1 CARROT RALLADA
1 GREEN PEPPER
COME TO TASTE

FOOD PYRAMID

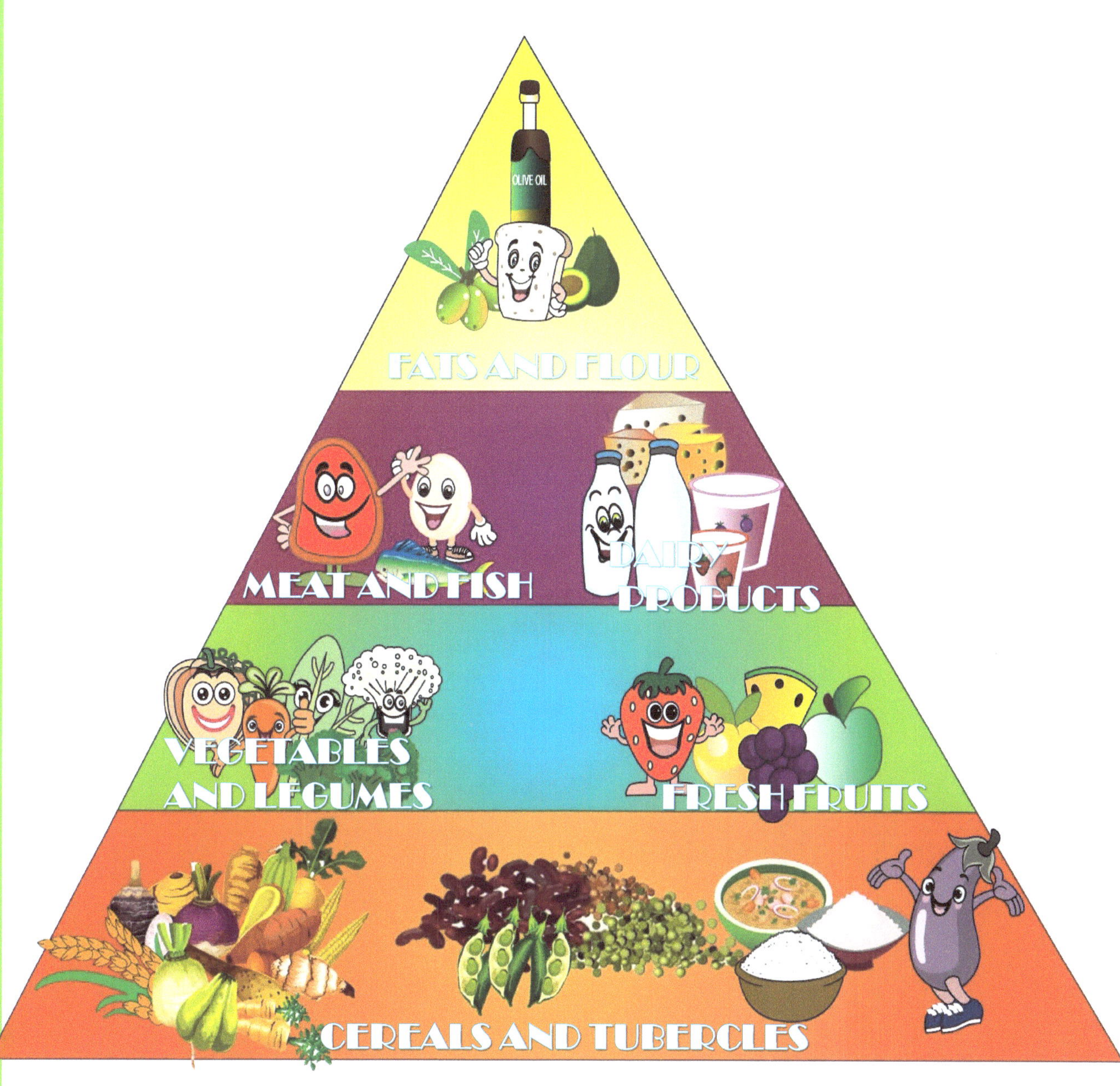

FOOD PYRAMID

Food	Recommended frequency	Weight per serving	Home Measurements
Bread, cereals, whole grains, rice, pasta, potatoes	4-6 servings/day (integral forms)	40-60 g bread 60-80 pasta, rice 150-200 g potatoes	3-4 slices or a bun 1 regular dish 1 large potato or two small
Milk and derivatives	2-4 servings/day	200-250 ml milk 200-250 g yogurt 40-60 g cured cheese 80-125 g fresh cheese	1 cup/cup milk 2 units yogurt 2-3 slices cheese 1 serving individually
Vegetables	2 servings/day	150-200 g	1 dish of varied salad 1 plate of cooked vegetables 1 large tomato, 2 carrots
Fruits	≥ 3 servings/day	120-200 g	1 medium piece 1 cup cherries, strawberries, 2 slices of melon
Olive oil	3-6 rations/day	day 10 ml	1 tablespoon
Vegetables	2-4 rations/Week	60-80 g	1 individual normal dish
Nuts	3-7 rations/Week	20-30 g	1 handful or individual ration
Fish and seafood	3-4 rations/Week	125-150 g	1 individual steak
Lean meats, birds	3-4 rations/week. Toggling your consumption	100-125 g	1 small steak 1 quarter chicken 1 quarter rabbit
Eggs	3-4 Rations/Week Middle	(53-63 g)	1-2 Eggs
Sausages and fat meats	Ocasional and moderate		
Sweets, snacks, soft drinks	Occasional and moderate		
Margarine, butter, pastries	Occasional and moderate		
Drinking water	4-8 rations/day	200 ml	1 glass or bottle
Wine/beer	Optional and moderate consumption		
Physical activity	Daily	30 minutes	

DIET TO LOSE WEIGHT WEEK 1

DIA 1

TIME	TIME OF DAY	AMOUNT	FOOD	
8 AM	BREAKFAST	1	Arepa	
		1	Cheese slice.	
		1	Coffee well	
		1/2	Milk cup	
		1	Glass of orange juice.	
11 AM	MID-MORNING	1	Mature mango	
		1	Glass with water	
1 PM	LUNCH	¼	Pound of pork	
		2	Lettuce leaves	
		1	Medium tomato	
		½	Red egg onion	
		1	Lemon	
		4	Rice spoons	
		1	Small well of green pea soup	
		1	Portion of dark chocolate	

TIME	SNACK	AMOUNT	FOOD	
3 PM	SNACK	6	Fresh Strawberries	
		1	Water cup	
4 PM	LIQUID	1	Glass of lemon juice	
5 PM	SNACK	1	Yogurt of any flavor unlike the fruit you've already eaten.	
7 PM	DINNER	1	Tuna can	
		2	Slices of bread	
		10	Spinach leaves	
		1	Cooked Carrot	
		3	Steamed Broccoli Flowers	
8 PM	DIGESTIVE	1	Hot chamomile tea cup	

DIET TO LOSE WEIGHT WEEK 1

DIA 2

TIME	TIME OF DAY	AMOUNT	FOOD	
8 AM	BREAKFAST	2 2 1 1	Slices of bread Eggs Hot Chocolate Grapefruit juice cup.	
11 AM	MID-MORNING	1 1	Orange Glass with water	
1 PM	LUNCH	¼ 10 1 ½ 2 1 1	Pound beef Spinach leaves Diced red pepper White Egg Onion Potato pure spoons Small bean soup puffin Portion of guava sandwich	

TIME	TIME OF DAY	AMOUNT	FOOD	
3 PM	SOMETHING	6 1	Blueberries Water cup	
4 PM	LIQUID	1	Glass of tree tomato juice	
5 PM	SNACK	1	Gelatin of any flavor unlike the fruit you've already eaten.	
7 PM	DINNER	1 2 1	Sardine can Slices of cooked cassava Portion of cabbage, carrot and lemon salad.	
8 PM	DIGESTIVE	1	Hot chamomile tea cup	

DIET TO LOSE WEIGHT

BREAKFAST

- Replace arepa with bread, oats, cheese bread, pandebono, omelets or two cooked potatoes.
- Replace the cheese with two eggs in your preferred style, or a sausage, or three strips of bacon.
- Replace coffee with tea, or chocolate.
- Don't stop drinking milk
-

MID-MORNING

Always consume a fruit at this time of the morning, hopefully different from the previous day.

We cannot forget that fiber consumption is totally necessary to improve our digestion.

We also can not forget the glass of water, which should be taken 15 minutes before the fruit.

The recommended amount of water daily is 8 glasses.

LUNCH

Reemplazar el ¼ de libra de carne de cerdo por carne de res, pollo, pescado, pavo, atún o ternera.

Comer cada día una ensalada diferente y variada que contenga lechuga, o repollo o espinacas, o coles, cebolla, pimientos verdes o rojos, coliflor o brócoli, o zanahoria, o espárragos.

EVENING

Replace rice with potato, corn, chickpeas, oats, pasta or bread.

Replace pea soup with lentil soup, bean soup of any kind, banana soup or potato soup.

Replace chocolate with a sweet dessert, butter biscuits etc.

DIET TO LOSE WEIGHT

SNACK

Replace strawberries with green, red or black grapes, blueberries or redberries, or two kiwis or bananas, or three small guavas, or three cherries, or six raspberries.

Drink a glass of water of 250 milliliters fifteen minutes before eating the fruit. If you don't have fluid retention problems, you can drink two glasses of water.

LIQUID

You can't stop drinking the glass of lemon juice at this time of day, because it's the one that will help you significantly improve your digestion, which will help you dilute the fats they include in your diet.

It should be taken with warm water, not hot, or cold.

SNACK

Replace yogurt with a gelatin of any flavor, preferably low in sugar or without sugar.

Every 8 days you can have a custard instead of yogurt or jelly.

DINNER

Replace the can of tuna with a can of sardine, 1/4-pound steamed salmon, one leg of roast chicken, two pork sausages, beef, turkey or veal. Replace the bread with four tablespoons of rice, or two cooked potatoes or a cooked cassava.

DIGESTIVE

Replace chamomile tea with fennel tea, anise or min.

LEARN HOW TO COMBINE FOOD

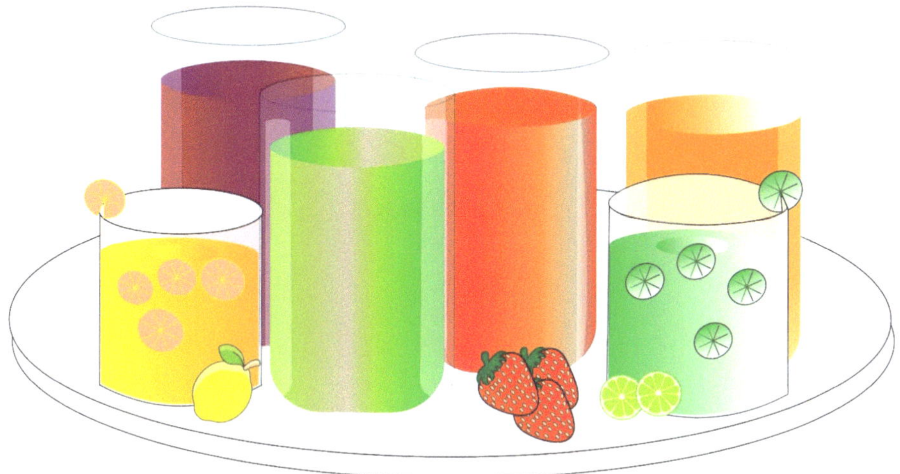

Foods are edible substances that are classified into proteins, carbohydrates (sugars, starches), fats (oils), mineral salts and vitamins.

It is recommended to consider the following before combining the food, to avoid fermentations that negatively affect our digestion and therefore our nutrition.

- ❖ If possible, take acids and starches in separate meals, because acids destroy the ptialine of saliva, which is where the first digestion of starches is done.
- ❖ Take proteins and starches in separate meals, because each causes a different activity in the digestive glands and we force the body to work double. Therefore some foods combined generate heavy and slow digestions.
- ❖ Take protein and acids at separate meals.
- ❖ Take fats and protein at separate meals.
- ❖ Drink sugars and protein in separate meals.
- ❖ Take starches and sugars at separate meals.
- ❖ It is recommended to consume melons and watermelons alone
- ❖ If possible, it is recommended to drink the milk alone
- ❖ Take the fruits alone, preferably in the mornings as breakfast.

Good digestion depends on the combinations of the foods we make. But as I told you before, it all depends on everyone. It's a matter of getting started and testing.

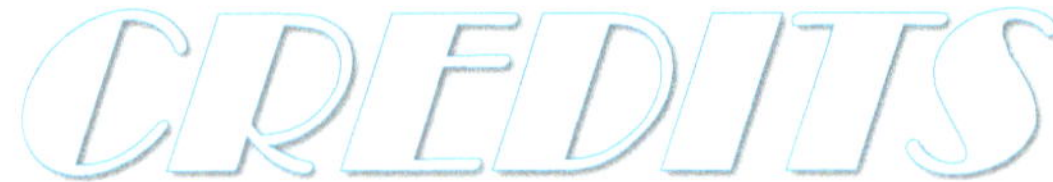

This research is based on research done on Wikipedia, in the book make your food your medicine of Dr. Colbert, specialist in Nutrition, from the book the combination of food by Dr. Herbert Shelton, specialist in dietetics, studies, in data extracted from the Spanish foundation of the heart and personal experiences throughout my existence.

Author: Gladys Yaneth Méndez Martinez